The Complete Keto Diet Cooking Guide

Low-carb dishes for a fit and healthy body

Ayla Newton

TABLE OF CONTENTS

techniques outlined in this book. By reading this document, the reader agrees that under no circumstances is the author responsible for any losses, 5 direct or indirect, which are incurred as a result of the use of information contained within this document, including, but not limited to, — errors, omissions, or inaccuracies.

BREAKFAST

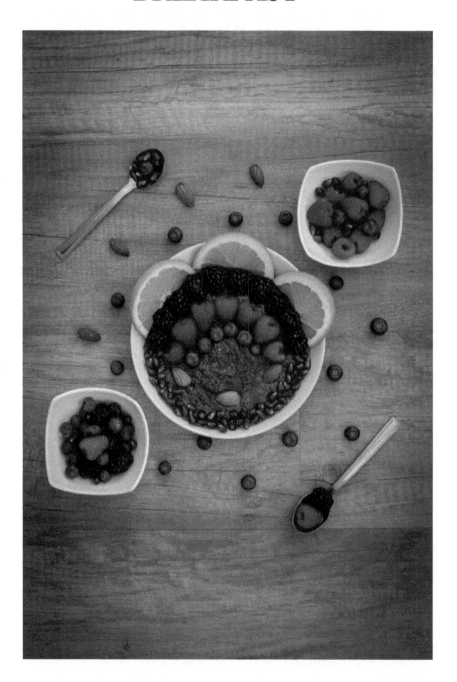

Fudge Oatmeal

Servings: 2

Preparation Time: 10 minutes

Ingredients:

- 1/3 cup: coconut milk -full-fat
- ½ cup: manitoba Harvest hemp hearts
- 1 tablespoon: sunflower butter
- 1 tablespoon: chia seed
- 2 tablespoon: cacao powder
- 3 drops: liquid stevia
- ½ teaspoon: vanilla extract
- Just a pinch: Himalayan rock salt -finely ground

Directions:

1. Combine all the ingredients in a jar and stir well.

2. Refrigerate covered overnight.

Nutritional Value:

478 Cal, 39.4 g total fat -17.9 g sat. fat, 128 mg sodium, 13.3 g carb., 8.8 g fiber, 18.6 g protein.

Creamy Hot Cocoa

Servings: 4

Preparation Time: 20 minutes

Cooking Time: 2 hours

Ingredients:

- ¼ cup + 2 tablespoon: unsweetened cocoa powder
- 8-10 packets: stevia
- ¼ teaspoon: salt
- 1 teaspoon: vanilla
- 3 cups: unsweetened almond milk
- ¼ cup: half and half

Directions:

1. Combine all the ingredients in a crockpot.

2. Cook covered for 2 hours on low, stirring occasionally.

3. Stir well.

Nutritional Value:

40 Cal, 5 g total fat -2 g sat. fat, 3 g net carb., 3g fiber, 3 g protein.

Maca Almond Smoothie

Servings: 1

Preparation Time: 5 minutes

Ingredients:

- ¾ cup: almond milk-unsweetened
- ¼ cup: coconut milk
- 1 tablespoon: almond butter -unsweetened
- 1 tablespoon: extra virgin coconut oil
- 1 tablespoon: collagen powder
- 2 teaspoon: maca powder

Directions:

1. Mix together all the ingredients in a blender.

2. Blend until smooth.

Nutritional Value:

500 Cal, 43.8 g total fat -25.5 g sat. fat, 10.9 g carb., 4.7g fiber, 14.6 g protein.

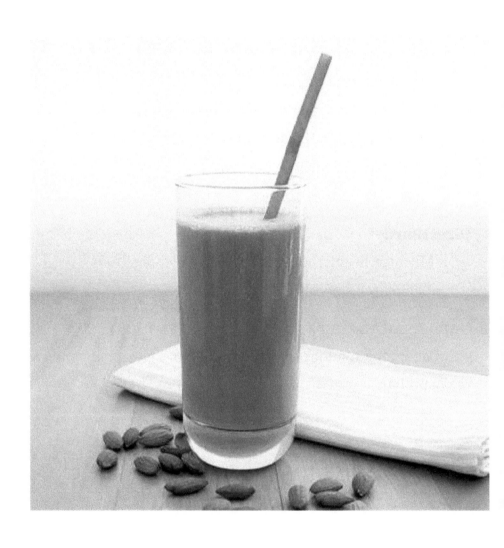

Nut Packed Coconut Granola

Servings: 20

Preparation Time: 5 minutes

Cooking Time: 28 minutes

Ingredients:

- Coconut flakes -unsweetened: ½ cup
- Raw almonds -slivered: 2 cups
- Raw pecans: 1 ¼ cup
- Raw walnuts: 1 cup
- Chia seeds: 3 tablespoon
- Flaxseed meal: 1 tablespoon
- Cinnamon -ground: 1 ½ teaspoon
- Coconut sugar: 2 tablespoon
- Sea salt: ¼ teaspoon
- Coconut oil: 3 tablespoon
- Maple syrup: ¼ cup + 1 tablespoon
- Dried blueberries: ¼ cup
- Roasted sunflower seeds -unsalted: ¼ cup

Directions:

1. Mix together the nuts, coconut, coconut sugar, cinnamon, flaxseed meal, and salt in a bowl.

2. Heat the coconut oil and maple syrup lightly in a saucepan over medium flame and pour it over the bowl's mixture.

3. Transfer the mixture onto a baking sheet, spreading it well, and bake in an oven preheated to 325 degrees Fahrenheit for 20 minutes.

4. Mix in the sunflower seeds and blueberries and bake at 340 degrees Fahrenheit for 5-8 minutes.

5. Remove and leave to cool.

Nutritional Value:

218 Cal, 18.5 g total fat -3.6 g sat. fat, 24 mg sodium, 10.6 g carb., 4.7g fiber, 6.2 g protein.

Choco-Green Smoothie

Servings: 2

Preparation Time: 5 minutes

Ingredients:

- Frozen berries: ½ cup
- Coconut cream: 1 cup
- Cocoa powder: ¼ cup
- Granulated sweetener: 1 tablespoon

Directions:

1. Combine all the ingredients in a high-speed blender.

2. Blend until smooth.

Nutritional Value:

186 Cal, 16.3 g total fat, 11.8 g carb., 6g fiber, 4.6 g protein.

BRUNCH

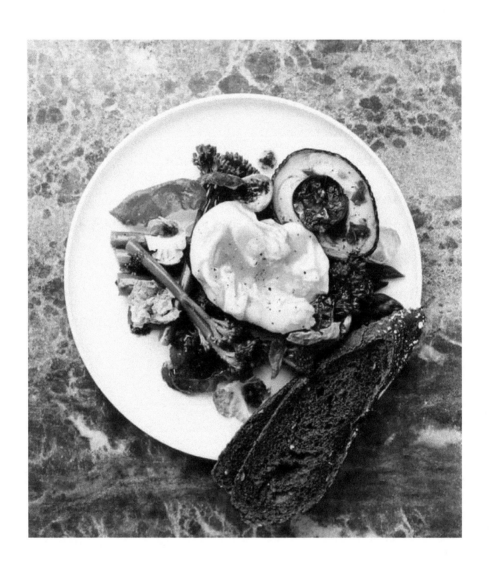

Avocado and Egg Salad

Servings: 2

Preparation Time: 15 minutes

Ingredients:

- 4 hard-boiled eggs
- 1 hass avocado
- 1/2 pack mixed leafy greens
- 1/2 cup vegetarian mayonnaise
- 2 cloves garlic, crushed
- 2 tsps. dijon mustard
- 1 tbsp. chives, chopped

Directions:

1. Hard boil the eggs by placing them in boiling water, letting them come back to a boil, and turning the heat off. Let stand, covered, for 12 minutes, then remove and cool.

2. Mix the mayo, garlic, and dijon in a small bowl. Stir to combine and season with salt and pepper.

3. Clean the salad greens, then dry and toss with the dressing. Cut the avocado in half, then remove the pit and slice both halves thinly. Place the avocado on top of the salad.

4. Cut the eggs into quarters and place them on the salad as a garnish. Finish with chives on the plate.

Nutritional Value Per Serving:

Net carbs: 6.1g, Protein: 17g, Fat: 36.3g, Calories: 436kcal.

Jelly & Peanut Butter Sandwiches

Servings: 4

Preparation Time: 5 minutes

Cooking Time: 2 minutes

Ingredients:

- Eggs - 2
- Almond flour: 3 tablespoon
- Coconut flour: 1 tablespoon
- Butter: 1 tablespoon
- Baking powder: ½ teaspoon
- Peanut butter: 1 tablespoon
- Jelly: ½ tablespoon

Directions:

1. Mix together all the ingredients except the butter and jelly in a mug.
2. Microwave for 2 minutes on high.
3. Remove and slice into 4 pieces.
4. Spread the butter on 2 slices and jelly on the other two.
5. Cover the butter slice with the jelly slice to make two sandwiches.

Nutritional Value:

498 Cal, 41 g total fat, 459 mg sodium, 14 g carbs, 6 g fiber, 22 g protein.

Chorizo and Mozzarella Omelet

Servings: 1

Cooking Time: 15 minutes

Ingredients

- 2 eggs
- 6 basil leaves
- 2 ounces mozzarella cheese
- 1 tbsp butter
- 1 tbsp water
- 4 thin slices of chorizo
- 1 tomato, sliced
- Salt and black pepper, to taste

Directions:

1. Whisk the eggs along with the water and some salt and pepper. Melt the butter in a skillet and cook the eggs for 30 seconds. Spread the chorizo slices over. Arrange the tomato and mozzarella over the chorizo. Cook for about 3 minutes. Cover the skillet and cook for 3 minutes until the omelet is set.

2. When ready, remove the pan from heat; run a spatula around the omelet's edges and flip it onto a warm plate, folded side down. Serve garnished with basil leaves and green salad.

Nutritional Value (Per Serving):

Kcal 451, Fat: 36.5g, Net Carbs: 3g, Protein: 30g

Tart with Broccoli & Greek Yogurt

Servings: 4

Cooking Time: 30 minutes

Ingredients

- 2 teaspoons olive oil
- 1 red onion, sliced
- 2 cups broccoli florets
- 2 garlic cloves, sliced
- Sea salt, black pepper, to taste
- 1/2 teaspoon paprika
- 1/4 teaspoon ground cumin
- 6 eggs
- 6 tablespoons Greek yogurt
- 1/2 cup cheddar cheese, shredded

Directions:

1. Heat the olive oil into an oven-safe pan over a moderate flame. Then, sauté the onion and broccoli until tender or about 3 minutes.

2. Then, add in the garlic and continue to sauté for 30 seconds more. Season with salt, black pepper, paprika, and cumin.

3. In a mixing dish, beat the eggs with the Greek yogurt until well combined. Pour the mixture into the pan and transfer it to the preheated oven.

4. Bake at 360 degrees F for about 18 minutes or until cooked through. Top with the cheese, switch to broil and let it cook for 5 minutes more. Bon appétit!

Nutritional Value (Per Serving):

308 Cal; 23.2g Fat; 5.3g Carbs; 19.2g Protein; 0.9g Fiber

Bacon Ranch Deviled Eggs

Servings: 2

Cooking Time: 0 minutes

Ingredients

- 1 slice of bacon, chopped, cooked
- 2/3 tsp ranch dressing
- 1 1/2 tbsp mayonnaise
- 1/3 tsp mustard paste
- 2 eggs, boiled
- Seasoning:
- ¼ tsp paprika

Directions:

1. Peel the boiled eggs, then slice in half lengthwise and transfer egg yolks to a medium bowl by using a spoon.

2. Mash the egg yolk, add remaining ingredients, except for bacon and paprika and stir until well combined.

3. Pipe the egg yolk mixture into egg whites, sprinkle with bacon and paprika and then serve.

Nutrition Info: 260 Calories; 24 g Fats; 8.9 g Protein; 0.6 g Net Carb; 0.1 g Fiber;

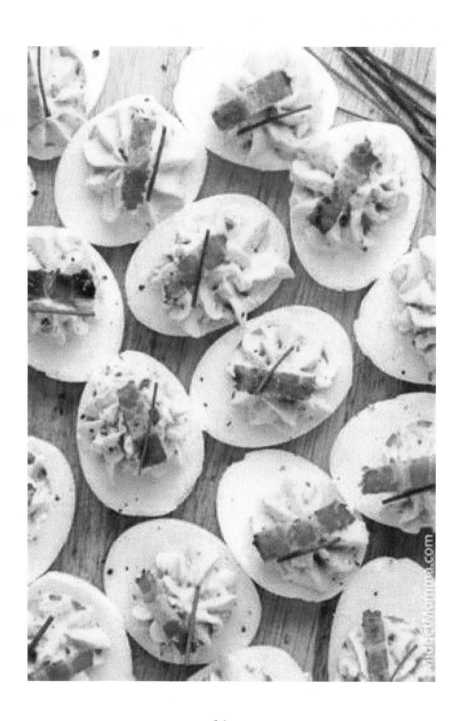

Pesto Deviled Eggs

Servings: 2

Cooking Time: 0 minutes

Ingredients

- 2 eggs, boiled
- 2 tbsp basil pesto
- 1 tbsp avocado oil

Directions:

1. Peel the boiled eggs, then slice in half lengthwise and transfer egg yolks to a medium bowl by using a spoon.

2. Mash the egg yolk, add remaining ingredients and stir until well combined.

3. Pipe the egg yolk mixture into egg whites and then serve.

Nutrition Info: 220 Calories; 19.2 g Fats; 8.1 g Protein; 1.7 g Net Carb; 1 g Fiber;

SOUP AND STEWS

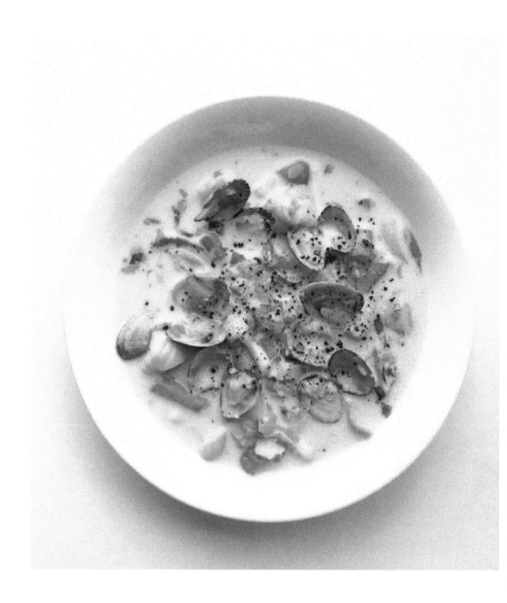

Hearty Fall Stew

Preparation Time: 15 minutes

Cooking Time: 8 hrs.

Servings: 6

Ingredients:

- tablespoons extra-virgin olive oil, divided
- 1 (2-pound/907-g) beef chuck roast, cut into 1-inch chunks
- 1/2 teaspoon salt
- 1/4 teaspoon freshly ground black pepper
- 1/4 cup apple cider vinegar
- 1/2 sweet onion, chopped
- 1 cup diced tomatoes
- teaspoon dried thyme
- 11/2 cups pumpkin, cut into 1-inch chunks
- 2 cups beef broth
- teaspoons minced garlic
- 1 tablespoon chopped fresh parsley, for garnish

Directions:

1. Add the beef to the skillet, and sprinkle salt and pepper to season. Cook the beef for 7 minutes or until well browned.

2. Put the cooked beef into the slow cooker and add the remaining ingredients, except for the parsley, to the slow cooker. Stir to mix well.

3. Slow cook for 8 hrs. and top with parsley before serving.

Nutritional Value:

Calories: 462 Fat: 19.1g Fiber: 11.6g Carbohydrates: 10.7 g Protein: 18.6 g

Chicken Mushroom Soup

Preparation Time: 15 minutes

Cooking Time: 10-15 minutes

Servings: 4

Ingredients:

- 6 cups of chicken stock
- 5 slices of chopped bacon
- 4 cups cooked chicken breast, chopped
- 3 cups of water
- 2 cups of chopped celery root
- 2 cups of sliced yellow squash
- 2 tablespoons of olive oil
- 1/2 teaspoon of avocado oil
- 1/4 cup of chopped basil
- 1/4 cup of chopped onion
- 1/4 cup of chopped tomatoes
- 1 tablespoon of ground garlic
- 1 cup of sliced white mushrooms
- 1 cup green beans
- Salt and black pepper

Directions:

1. Heat oil in a skillet, add in half of the onions, sauté until soft. Put in bacon and fry for a minute and a half.

2. Then, add in onions, garlic, tomatoes, and mushrooms, stir fry for three minutes.

3. Put in stock and fat water with the rest of the ingredients. Let it simmer for 10-15 minutes. Serve hot.

Nutritional Value:

Calories: 268 Fat: 10.5g Fiber: 4.9g Carbohydrates: 3.1 g Protein: 12.9g

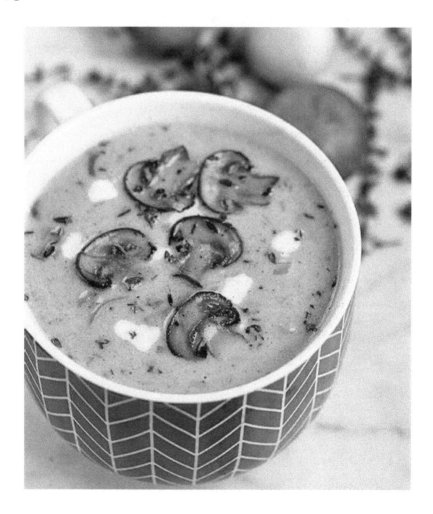

Cold Green Beans and Avocado Soup

Preparation Time: 15 minutes

Cooking Time: 15 minutes

Servings: 4

Ingredients:

- tbsp. butter
- tbsp. almond oil
- 1 garlic clove, minced
- 1 cup (227 g) green beans (fresh or frozen)
- 1/4 avocado
- 1 cup heavy cream
- 1/2 cup grated cheddar cheese + extra for garnish
- 1/2 tsp. coconut aminos
- Salt to taste

Directions:

1. Heat the butter and almond oil in a large skillet and sauté the garlic for 30 seconds.
2. Add the green beans and stir-fry for 10 minutes or until tender.
3. Add the mixture to a food processor and top with the avocado, heavy cream, cheddar cheese, coconut aminos, and salt.
4. Blend the ingredients until smooth.

5. Pour the soup into serving bowls, cover with plastic wraps and chill in the fridge for at least 2 hours.

6. Enjoy afterward with a garnish of grated white sharp cheddar cheese.

Nutritional Value:

Calories: 301 Fat: 3.1g Fiber: 11.5g Carbohydrates: 2.8 g Protein: 3.1g

Creamy Mixed Seafood Soup

Preparation Time: 15 minutes

Cooking Time: 15 minutes

Servings: 4

Ingredients:

- tbsp. avocado oil
- garlic cloves, minced
- 3/4 tbsp. almond flour
- 1 cup vegetable broth
- 1 tsp. dried dill
- lb. frozen mixed seafood
- Salt and black pepper to taste
- 1 tbsp. plain vinegar
- cups cooking cream
- Fresh dill leaves to garnish

Directions:

1. Heat oil sauté the garlic for 30 seconds or until fragrant.

2. Stir in the almond flour until brown.

3. Mix in the vegetable broth until smooth and stir in the dill, seafood mix, salt, and black pepper.

4. Bring the soup to a boil and then simmer for 3 to 4 minutes or until the seafood cooks.

5. Add the vinegar, cooking cream, and stir well. Garnish with dill, serve.

Nutritional Value:

Calories: 361 Fat: 12.4g Fiber: 8.5g Carbohydrates:3.9 g Protein:
11.7g

Roasted Tomato and Cheddar Soup

Preparation Time: 10 minutes

Cooking Time: 15-20 minutes

Servings: 4

Ingredients:

- 2 tbsp. butter
- 2 medium yellow onions, sliced
- 4 garlic cloves, minced
- 5 thyme sprigs
- 8 basil leaves + extra for garnish
- 8 tomatoes
- 1/2 tsp. red chili flakes
- 2 cups vegetable broth
- Salt and black pepper to taste
- 1 cup grated cheddar cheese (white and sharp)

Directions:

1. Melt the butter in a pot and sauté the onions and garlic for 3 minutes or until softened.
2. Stir in the thyme, basil, tomatoes, red chili flakes, and vegetable broth. Season with salt and black pepper.
3. Boil it, then simmer for 10 minutes or until the tomatoes soften. Puree all ingredients until smooth. Season.
4. Garnish with the cheddar cheese and basil. Serve warm.

Nutritional Value:

Calories: 341 Fat: 12.9g Fiber: 9.6g Carbohydrates: 4.8 g Protein: 4.1g

MAIN

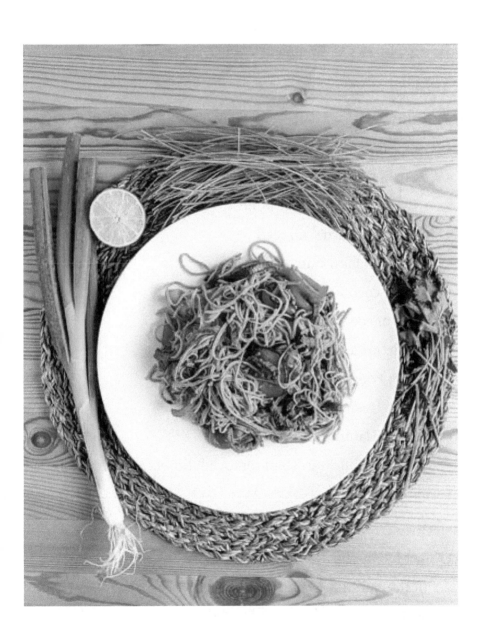

Eggplant and Coconut Milk Curry with Cauliflower "Rice"

Preparation Time: 10 minutes

Cooking Time: 25 minutes

Servings: 4

Ingredients:

- 1 lb. eggplant: skin on and cut into 1-inch pieces
- ½ white onion: diced
- 1-inch piece of ginger: minced
- 2 cloves of garlic: minced
- ½ cup Cashew nuts
- 3 tbsp. coconut oil
- 1 cup of coconut milk
- 1 tbsp. mild curry powder
- Salt & Pepper to taste
- ½ cup fresh coriander: roughly chopped
- For the Cauliflower "Rice":
- 1 large cauliflower: stem removed, florets cut into medium pieces

Directions:

1. Start by making the cauliflower "Rice."

2. Put the cauliflower florets in a food processor with a grating blade. A regular blade will also do.

3. Pulse until the cauliflower looks like rice. Make sure not to overdo or you will end up with a mash.

4. If you do not have a food processor, you can use a hand grater.

5. Set the rice aside.

6. Put the coconut oil in a large frying pan and heat over medium-high heat.

7. When the oil is hot, add the eggplant and cook for approximately 5 minutes until the eggplant is seared. Stir occasionally.

8. Add onion, garlic, ginger, and cook until soft while stirring.

9. You can add a little bit more oil if necessary, as the eggplant tends to absorb most of it.

10. Add curry powder and stir well.

11. After about 1 minute, add cashew nuts, coconut milk, black pepper, and salt pinch.

12. Simmer for about 5 minutes or until the sauce is slightly reduced.

13. Take off the heat and add fresh coriander. Stir gently.

14. Serve over the cauliflower "Rice."

Pan-Seared Tempeh Steak with Roasted Cabbage and Walnuts

Preparation Time: 1 hour

Cooking Time: 40 minutes

Servings: 4

Ingredients:

For the Pan-Seared Tempeh:

- 1 lb. tempeh: cut into 3 ½ inches long by 3/8 inch thick slices
- ¼ cup of water
- 1 garlic clove: minced
- 1 tsp. dried oregano
- ¼ tsp. pepper flakes
- ¾ cup extra virgin olive oil
- 6 tbsp. red wine vinegar

For the Roasted Cabbage:

- 1 medium head of green cabbage: cut into 8 wedges and core trimmed.
- Juice of 1 lemon
- 2 tbsp. extra virgin olive oil
- Salt & Pepper

Directions:

1. Preheat oven to 450F.

2. In a plastic sealable bag, combine the water, red wine vinegar, garlic, oregano, and pepper flakes. Add tempeh, press out the air, and seal the bag.

3. Toss the bag to coat the tempeh with the marinade completely.

4. If you do not have a sealable bag, you can use a mixing ball and cover it with cling film.

5. Refrigerate your tempeh for 1 hour. You can marinate for longer if you have time.

6. Place wedges on a roasting tray. Arrange them in a single layer.

7. Sprinkle walnuts on top.

8. In a small bowl, whisk together the extra virgin olive oil and lemon juice.

9. Pour the mixture on top of the cabbage and season with salt and pepper to taste.

10. Gently toss the wedges to coat with the mixture completely.

11. Roast each side of the cabbage for approximately 15 minutes until nicely browned.

12. After 1 hour, remove tempeh from the marinade.

13. Pat tempeh dry with a piece of paper towel.

14. Take a large skillet or frying pan and heat the olive oil over medium heat.

15. When the oil is hot, add tempeh and cook for about 2-4 minutes until golden brown.

16. Turn tempeh on the other side and reduce heat. Cook for another 2-4 minutes.

17. Remove from the heat and move tempeh onto a sheet of paper towel over a plate.

18. Serve on a plate with the cabbage.

19. You can top with a drizzle of extra virgin olive oil and pepper.

20. Serve topped with lots of avocados and garnish with pumpkin seeds.

Edamame Kelp Noodles

Servings: 2

Preparation Time: 10 minutes

Cooking Time: 10 minutes

Ingredients:

- Kelp noodles: 1 package
- Carrots -julienned: ¼ cup
- Edamame -shelled: ½ cup
- Mushrooms -sliced: ¼ cup
- Frozen spinach: 1 cup

Sauce:

- Tamari: 2 tablespoon
- Sesame oil: 1 tablespoon
- Ground ginger: ½ teaspoon
- Garlic powder - ½ teaspoon
- Sriracha: ¼ teaspoon

Directions:

1. Soak the kelp noodles in water and then drain.
2. Place the sauce ingredients in a saucepan over medium flame and then toss in the veggies.
3. Once warm, add in the noodles.
4. Simmer covered for a few minutes, stirring occasionally.

Nutritional Value:

139 Cal, 8.6 g total fat, 4.9 g net carbs, 4.5g fiber, 7.8 g protein.

Pecan Sweet Potato casserole

Servings: 8

Preparation Time: 20 minutes

Cooking Time: 50 minutes

Ingredients:

- Butternut squash -peeled, cubed: 4 cups
- Cauliflower -separated into florets: 1
- Butter -melted: 2 tablespoon
- Garlic salt: ¾ teaspoon
- Cinnamon: 1 teaspoon
- Black pepper: ½ teaspoon
- Sweetener of choice: 4 teaspoon

- Topping:
- Pecans: 2 cups
- Sweetener of choice: 1/3 cup
- Cinnamon: 1 teaspoon
- Butter: 2 tablespoon
- Garlic salt: 1/8 teaspoon

Directions:

1. Toss together all the ingredients apart from the topping and spread it on a baking sheet lined with foil and greased lightly, leaving aside a tablespoon of butter and the sweetener.

2. Roast for 30-35 minutes in an oven preheated to 400 degrees Fahrenheit, tossing the veggies halfway through.

3. Puree the vegetables in the food processor and transfer them into a casserole dish, mixing in the remaining butter and sweetener.

4. Even out the top and spread the pecan topping over.

5. Roast for 20 minutes in the oven until the top becomes golden.

Nutritional Value:

293 Cal, 26 g total fat -5 g sat. fat, 16 mg chol., 26 mg sodium, 17 g carbs, 7g fiber, 5 g protein.

Keto Soufflé

Preparation Time: 27 minutes

Servings: 6

Ingredients:

- 2 eggs
- 2-ounce softened cream cheese
- 1 cup sharp cheddar cheese
- ½ cup Asiago cheese
- ½ cup plain yogurt
- 2 tbsp. heavy cream
- 1 chopped head cauliflower
- ¼ cup minced fresh chives
- 2 tbsp. softened butter

Directions:

1. Grease 1¼ quart casserole dish that will fit in an Instant Pot. Keep aside.

2. In a food processor, add eggs, cream cheese, cheddar cheese, Asiago cheese, yogurt, and heavy cream and pulse until smooth and frothy.

3. Add cauliflower and pulse until chunky.

4. Gently fold in chives and butter.

5. Transfer the mixture to the prepared casserole dish.

6. In the bottom of the Instant Pot, arrange a steamer trivet and pour 1 cup of water.

7. Place the casserole dish on top of the trivet.

8. Secure the lid and place the pressure valve in the "Seal" position.

9. Select "Manual" and cook under "High Pressure" for about 12 minutes.

10. Select the "Cancel" and carefully do a "Natural" release for about 10 minutes and then do a "Quick" release.

11. Remove the lid and serve.

Nutrition Values:

Calories 234, Total Fat 17.5g, Net Carbs 1.48g, Protein 11.7g, Fiber 3.1g

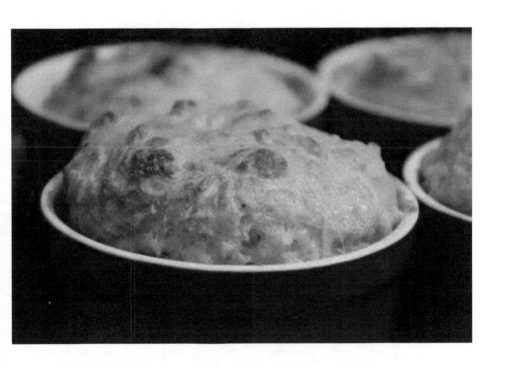

MEAT

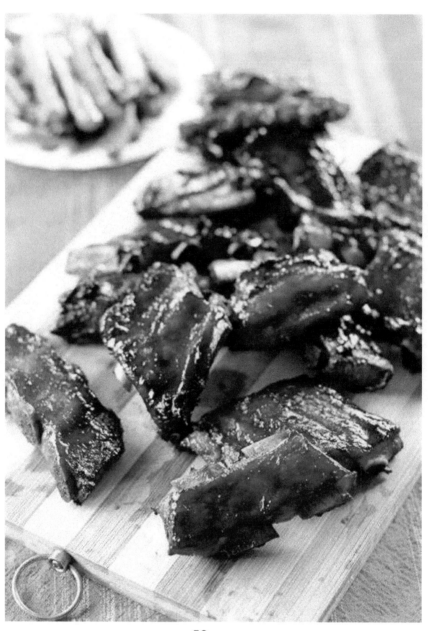

Beef Wellington

Preparation Time: 20 minutes

Cooking Time: 40 minutes

Servings: 4

Ingredients:

- (4-ounce) grass-fed beef tenderloin steaks, halved
- Salt, and ground black pepper, as required
- 1 tablespoon butter
- 1 cup mozzarella cheese, shredded
- 1/2 cup almond flour
- 4 tablespoons liver pate

Directions:

1. Preheat your oven to 400°F. Grease a baking sheet.
2. Season the steaks with pepper and salt.
3. Sear the beef steaks for about 2–3 minutes per side.
4. In a microwave-safe bowl, add the mozzarella cheese and microwave for about 1 minute.
5. Remove from the microwave and stir in the almond flour until a dough forms.
6. Place the dough between 2 parchment paper pieces and, with a rolling pin, roll to flatten it.
7. Remove the upper parchment paper piece. Divide the rolled dough into four pieces.

8. Place one tablespoon of pate onto each dough piece and top with one steak piece.

9. Cover each steak piece with dough completely.

10. Arrange the covered steak pieces onto the prepared baking sheet in a single layer.

11. Baking time: 20-30 minutes Serve warm.

Nutritional Value:

Calories: 412 Fat: 15.6g Fiber: 9.1g Carbohydrates: 4.9 g Protein: 18.5g

Sticky Pork Ribs

Preparation Time: 25 minutes

Cooking Time: 90 minutes

Servings: 8

Ingredients:

- 1/4 cups granulated erythritol
- 1 tablespoon garlic powder
- 1 tablespoon paprika
- 1/2 teaspoon red chili powder
- 4 pounds pork ribs, membrane removed
- Salt and ground black pepper, as required
- 11/2 teaspoons liquid smoke
- 11/2 cups sugar-free BBQ sauce

Directions:

1. Preheat your oven to 300° F.

2. In a bowl, mix well erythritol, garlic powder, paprika, and chili powder. Season the ribs with pepper and salt. And then coat with the liquid smoke. Now, rub the ribs evenly with erythritol mixture.

3. Arrange ribs onto the prepared baking sheet, meaty side down.

4. Arrange two layers of foil on top of ribs and then roll and crimp edges tightly.

5. Bake for about 2–21/2 hours or until the desired doneness. Now, set the oven to broiler.

6. With a sharp knife, cut the ribs into serving-sized portions and evenly coat with the barbecue sauce.

7. Arrange the ribs onto a broiler pan, bony side up. Broil for about 1–2 minutes per side.

8. Remove from the oven and serve hot.

Nutritional Value:

Calories: 415 Fat: 18.1g Fiber: 12.5g Carbohydrates: 3.1 g Protein: 18.5g

Creamy Pork and Celeriac Gratin

Preparation Time: 20 minutes

Cooking Time: 60 minutes

Servings: 4

Ingredients:

- 1/2 lb. celeriac, peeled and thinly sliced
- 1/3 cup almond milk
- 1/2 cup heavy cream
- 1/4 tsp. nutmeg powder
- Salt and black pepper to taste
- 1 tbsp. olive oil
- 1 lb. ground pork
- 1/2 medium white onion, chopped
- 1 garlic clove, minced
- 1/2 tsp. unsweetened tomato paste
- 3 tbsp. butter for greasing
- 1 cup crumbled queso fresco cheese
- 1 tbsp. chopped fresh parsley for garnish

Directions:

1. Let the oven preheat to 375° F.

2. In a saucepan, add the celeriac, almond milk, heavy cream, nutmeg powder, and salt.

3. Cook until the celeriac softens. Drain afterward and set aside.

4. Heat oil and cook the pork for 5 minutes or starting to brown—season with salt and black pepper.

5. Stir in the onion, garlic, and cook for 5 minutes or until the onions soften. The tomato paste must be added and continue cooking.

6. Grease a baking dish and lay half of the celeriac on the bottom of the dish. Spread the tomato-pork sauce on top and cover with the remaining celeriac. Finish the topping with the queso fresco cheese.

7. Let the gratin bake for about 45 minutes or until the cheese melts and is golden brown.

8. Remove from the oven to cool for 5 to 10 minutes, garnish with the parsley, and serve afterward.

Nutritional Value:

Calories: 486 Fat: 19.4g Fiber: 10.3g Carbohydrates: 8.5 g Protein: 19.2 g

BBQ Pulled Beef

Preparation Time: 15 minutes

Cooking Time: 6 hrs.

Servings: 10

Ingredients:

- 3 lbs. boneless chuck roast
- 2 tablespoons of salt
- 2 tablespoon of garlic powder
- 1 tablespoon of onion powder
- 1/4 apple cider vinegar
- 2 tablespoons of coconut aminos
- 1/2 cup of bone broth
- 1/4 cup of melted butter
- 1 tablespoon of black pepper
- 1 tablespoon of smoked paprika
- 2 tablespoons of tomato paste

Directions:

1. Mix salt, onion, paprika, black pepper, and garlic.

2. Next is to rub the mixture on the beef and then put the beef in a slow cooker

3. Use another bowl to melt butter. Then, add tomato paste, coconut aminos, and vinegar.

4. Pour it all over the beef. Next is to add the bone broth into the slow cooker by pouring it around the beef

5. Cook for about 6 hrs.

6. After that, take out the beef and increase the cooker's temperature so that the sauce can thicken. Tear the beef before adding it to the slow cooker and toss with the sauce.

Nutritional Value:

Calories: 315 Fat: 17g Fiber: 11.9g Carbohydrates: 4.1 g Protein: 18.9g

Nut-Stuffed Pork Chops

Preparation Time: 20 minutes

Cooking Time: 30 minutes

Servings: 4

Ingredients:

- ounces goat cheese
- 1/2 cup chopped walnuts
- 1/4 cup toasted chopped almonds
- 1 teaspoon chopped fresh thyme
- center-cut pork chops, butterflied
- Sea salt
- Freshly ground black pepper
- 2 tablespoons olive oil

Directions:

1. Preheat the oven to 400° F.

2. In a container, stir together the goat cheese, walnuts, almonds, and thyme until well mixed.

3. Season the pork chops inside and outside with salt and pepper. Stuff each chop, pushing the filling to the bottom of the cut section. Secure the stuffing with toothpicks through the meat.

4. Heat oil. Pan sear the pork chops until they're browned on each side, about 10 minutes in total.

5. Cooked through about 20 minutes. Serve after removing the toothpicks.

Nutritional Value:

Calories: 425 Fat: 19.5g Fiber: 7.9g Carbohydrates:6.5 g Protein: 19.4g

Roasted Pork Loin with Brown Mustard Sauce

Preparation Time: 10 minutes

Cooking Time: 70 minutes

Servings: 8

Ingredients:

- 1 (2-pound) boneless pork loin roast
- Sea salt
- Freshly ground black pepper
- 3 tablespoons olive oil
- 11/2 cups decadent (whipping) cream
- 3 tablespoons grainy mustard, such as Pommery

Directions:

1. Preheat the oven to 375° F.
2. Season the pork roast all over with sea salt and pepper.
3. Heat oil, then all the roast sides must be browned, about 6 minutes in total, and place the roast in a baking dish.
4. When there are approximately 15 minutes of roasting time left, place a small saucepan over medium heat and add the heavy cream and mustard.
5. Stir the sauce until it simmers, then reduce the heat to low. Simmer the sauce until it is vibrant and thick, about 5 minutes. Remove the pan from the heat and set aside.

Nutritional Value:

Calories: 415 Fat: 18.4g Fiber: 11.3g Carbohydrates: 3.1 g Protein: 17.4g

Lamb Chops with Tapenade

Preparation Time: 15 minutes

Cooking Time: 25 minutes

Servings: 4

Ingredients:

FOR THE TAPENADE

- cup pitted Kalamata olive
- tablespoons chopped fresh parsley
- 2 tablespoons extra-virgin olive oil
- 2 teaspoons minced garlic
- 2 teaspoons freshly squeezed lemon juice

FOR THE LAMB CHOPS

- 2 (1-pound) racks French-cut lamb chops (8 bones each)
- Sea salt
- Freshly ground black pepper
- 1 tablespoon olive oil

Directions:

TO MAKE THE TAPENADE

1. Place the olives, parsley, olive oil, garlic, and lemon juice in a food processor and process until the mixture is puréed, but still slightly chunky.

2. Transfer the tapenade to a container and store it sealed in the refrigerator until needed.

TO MAKE THE LAMB CHOPS

1. Preheat the oven to 450° F.

2. Season the lamb racks with pepper and salt Heat oil

3. Pan sear the lamb racks on all sides until browned, about 5 minutes in total.

4. Arrange the racks upright in the skillet, with the bones interlaced, and roast them for about 20 minutes for medium-rare or until the internal temperature reaches 125° F.

Nutritional Value:

Calories: 387 Fat: 17.4g Fiber: 12.1g Carbohydrates: 5.4 g Protein: 18.9g

Sesame Pork with Green Beans

Preparation Time: 5 minutes

Cooking Time: 10 minutes

Servings: 2

Ingredients:

- 2 boneless pork chops
- Pink Himalayan salt
- Freshly ground black pepper
- 2 tablespoons toasted sesame oil, divided
- 2 tablespoons soy sauce
- 1 teaspoon Sriracha sauce
- 1 cup fresh green beans

Directions:

1. On a cutting board, pat the pork chops dry with a paper towel. Slice the chops into strips and season with pink Himalayan salt and pepper.

2. In a large skillet over medium heat, heat one tablespoon of sesame oil. Add the pork strips and cook them for 7 minutes, stirring occasionally.

3. In a small bowl, mix the remaining one tablespoon of sesame oil, the soy sauce, and the Sriracha sauce. Pour into the skillet with the pork.

4. Add the green beans to the skillet, reduce the heat to medium-low, and simmer for 3 to 5 minutes.

5. Divide the pork, green beans, and sauce between two wide, shallow bowls and serve.

Nutritional Value:

Calories: 387 Fat: 15.1g Fiber: 10g Carbohydrates: 4.1 g Protein: 18.1 g

POULTRY

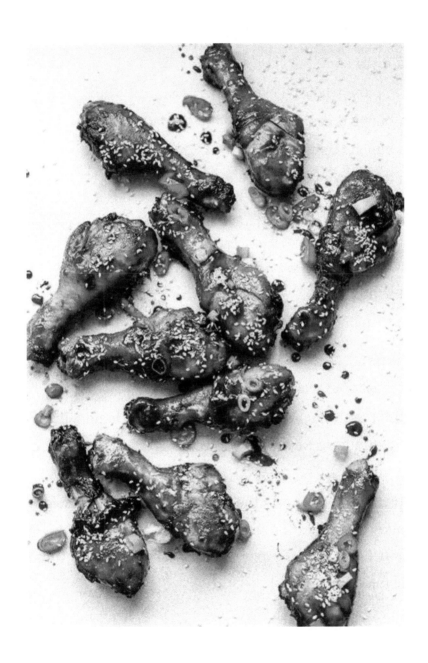

Roast Chicken with Herb Stuffing

Servings: 8

Cooking Time: 120 minutes

Ingredients

- 5-pound whole chicken
- 1 bunch oregano
- 1 bunch thyme
- 1 tbsp marjoram
- 1 tbsp parsley
- 1 tbsp olive oil
- 2 pounds Brussels sprouts
- 1 lemon
- 4 tbsp butter

Directions:

1. Preheat your oven to 450° F.

2. Stuff the chicken with oregano, thyme, and lemon. Roast for 15 minutes. Reduce the heat to 3°F and cook for 40 minutes.

3. Spread the butter over the chicken, and sprinkle parsley and marjoram. Add the brussels sprouts. Return to the oven and bake for 40 more minutes. Let sit for 10 minutes before carving.

Nutritional Value (Per Serving):

Kcal 432, Fat: 32g, Net Carbs: 5.1g, Protein: 30g

One Pot Chicken with Mushrooms

Servings: 6

Cooking Time: 35 minutes

Ingredients

- 2 cups sliced mushrooms
- ½ tsp onion powder
- ½ tsp garlic powder
- ¼ cup butter
- 1 tsp Dijon mustard
- 1 tbsp tarragon, chopped
- 2 pounds chicken thighs
- Salt and black pepper, to taste

Directions:

1. Season the thighs with salt, pepper, garlic, and onion powder. Melt the butter in a skillet, and cook the chicken until browned; set aside. Add mushrooms to the same fat and cook for about 5 minutes.

2. Stir in Dijon mustard and ½ cup of water. Return the chicken to the skillet. Season to taste with salt and pepper, reduce the heat and cover, and let simmer for 15 minutes. Stir in tarragon. Serve warm.

Nutritional Value (Per Serving): Kcal 447, Fat: 37g, Net Carbs: 1g, Protein: 31g

Herb Roasted Chicken Drumsticks

Servings: 2

Cooking Time: 12 minutes

Ingredients

- 2 chicken drumsticks
- ¼ of a lime, juiced
- ½ tsp Italian herb blend
- ½ tsp garlic powder
- 2 tbsp avocado oil

Seasoning:

- 1/3 tsp salt

Directions:

1. Turn on the oven, then set it to 400 degrees F and let it preheat. Meanwhile, place chicken into a bowl and add remaining ingredients except for oil and toss until well-coated.

2. Transfer chicken drumsticks into a baking sheet greased with avocado oil and then bake for 12 minutes until cooked and slightly crispy, turning halfway. Serve.

Nutritional Value:

377 Calories; 27 g Fats; 27 g Protein; 4 g Net Carb; 1 g Fiber;

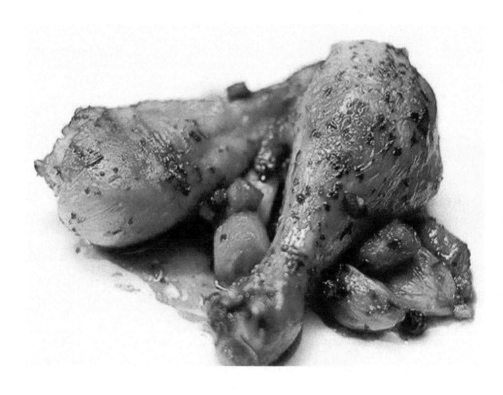

Chicken Parmigiana

Servings: 4

Cooking Time: 26 minutes

Ingredients

- 1 large organic egg, beaten
- ½ cup of superfine blanched almond flour
- ¼ cup Parmesan cheese, grated
- ½ teaspoon dried parsley
- ½ teaspoon paprika
- ½ teaspoon garlic powder
- Salt and ground black pepper, as required
- 4 6-ounces grass-fed skinless, boneless chicken breasts, pounded into the ½-inch thickness
- ¼ cup olive oil1½ cups marinara sauce
- 4 ounces mozzarella cheese, thinly sliced
- 2 tablespoons fresh parsley, chopped

Directions:

1. Preheat the oven to 375 degrees F. Add the beaten egg into a shallow dish.

2. Place the almond flour, Parmesan, parsley, spices, salt, and black pepper in another shallow dish and mix well.

3. Dip each chicken breast into the beaten egg and then coat with the flour mixture.

4. Heat the oil in a deep skillet over medium-high heat and fry the chicken breasts for about 3 minutes per side.

5. With a slotted spoon, transfer the chicken breasts onto a paper towel-lined plate to drain.

6. In the bottom of a casserole dish, place about ½ cup of marinara sauce and spread evenly.

7. Arrange the chicken breasts over marinara sauce in a single layer.

8. Top with the remaining marinara sauce, followed by mozzarella cheese slices.

9. Bake for about 20 minutes or until done completely.

10. Remove from the oven and serve hot with the garnishing of fresh parsley.

Nutritional Value (Per Serving): Calories: 542; Net Carbs: 5.7g; Carbohydrate: 9g; Fiber: 3.3g; Protein: 54.2g; Fat: 33.2g; Sugar: 3.8g; Sodium: 609mg

FISH

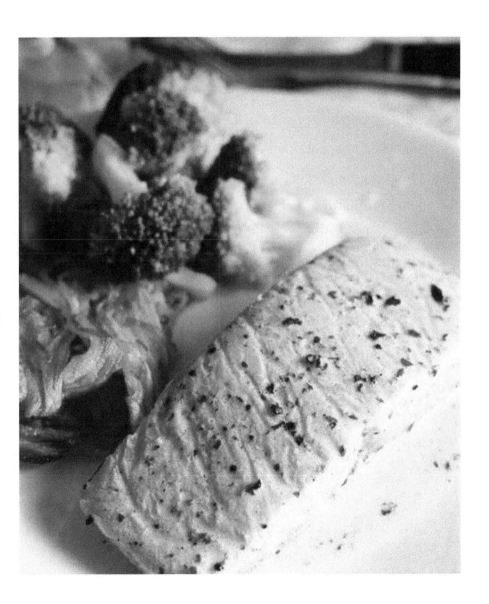

Traditional Salmon Panzanella

Servings: 4

Cooking Time: 25 minutes

Ingredients

- 1 lb skinned salmon, cut into 4 steaks each
- 1 cucumber, cubed
- Salt and black pepper to taste
- 8 black olives, chopped
- 1 tbsp capers, rinsed
- 2 large tomatoes, diced
- 3 tbsp white wine vinegar
- ¼ cup thinly sliced red onion
- 3 tbsp olive oil
- 2 slices zero carb bread, cubed
- ¼ cup sliced basil leaves

Directions:

1. Preheat grill to 360 F. In a bowl, mix cucumbers, olives, pepper, capers, tomatoes, wine vinegar, onion, olive oil, bread, and basil leaves.

2. Let sit for the flavors to incorporate. Season the salmon with salt, then grill them on both sides for 8 minutes.

3. Serve the salmon steaks warm on a bed of the veggies salad.

Nutritional Value (Per Serving): Cal 338; Net Carbs 3.1g; Fat 21g; Protein 28.5g

Tuna Zoodle Casserole

Servings: 2

Cooking Time: 20 minutes

Ingredients

- 1 zucchini5 oz tuna, packed in water, drained
- 4 tbsp whipping cream
- 3 tbsp grated cheddar cheese
- 4 oz almond milk, unsweetened

Seasoning:

- 1 tbsp butter, unsalted
- ½ tsp garlic powder
- 2 oz of chicken bone broth

Directions:

1. Turn on the oven, then set it to 350 degrees F and let it preheat. Cut zucchini into noodles, spread them on a baking sheet, and then bake for 5 minutes or more until moisture has evaporated completely, stirring every 5 minutes.

2. Meanwhile, take a medium skillet pan, place it over medium heat, add butter and when it melts, add garlic powder, cream, broth, and tbsp cheddar cheese, stir until smooth and cook for 2 minutes until cheese has melted.

3. Add tuna, stir until combined, and then remove the pan from heat. Take a casserole dish, spread half of the pre-

baked zucchini noodles in its bottom, top with half of the tuna mixture, cover with remaining zucchini noodles, and then spread the remaining tuna mixture on it. Sprinkle remaining cheese on top and then bake for 12 to 15 minutes until cheese has melted and the mixture is bubbling. Serve.

Nutritional Value:

320 Calories; 21.2 g Fats; 24.3 g Protein; 4.7 g Net Carb; 1.6 g Fiber;

Trout and Mustard Sauce

Servings: 4

Cooking Time: 20 minutes

Ingredients

- 2 tablespoons olive oil
- 2 garlic cloves, minced
- 2 spring onions, chopped
- 4 trout fillets, boneless
- A pinch of salt and black pepper
- 2 tablespoons Dijon mustard
- Juice and zest of 1 lime
- ½ cup heavy cream
- 2 tablespoons chives, chopped

Directions:

1. Heat up a pan and put oil over medium heat; add the garlic and the spring onions, stir and sauté for 3 minutes.
2. Add the fish and cook it for 4 minutes on each side. Add the mustard and the other ingredients, toss gently, cook over medium heat for 10 minutes more, divide between plates and serve.

Nutritional Value:

calories 171, fat 5, fiber 1, carbs 6, protein 23

Dilled Salmon in Creamy Sauce

Servings: 2

Cooking Time: 15 minutes

Ingredients

- 2 salmon fillets
- ¾ tsp dried tarragon
- 2 tbsp olive oil
- ¾ tsp dried dill

Sauce:

- 2 tbsp butter
- ½ tsp dill
- ½ tsp tarragon
- ¼ cup heavy cream
- Salt and black pepper to taste

Directions:

1. Season the salmon with dill and tarragon. Put the olive oil in a pan over medium heat. Add salmon and cook for about 4 minutes on both sides. Set aside.

2. Sauce making: melt the butter and add the dill and tarragon. Cook for 30 seconds to infuse the flavors. Whisk in the cream, season with salt and black pepper, and cook for 3 minutes. Serve the salmon topped with the sauce.

Nutritional Value (Per Serving): Kcal 468, Fat: 40g, Net Carbs: 1.5g, Protein:22g

Saucy Salmon in Tarragon Sauce

Servings: 2

Cooking Time: 20 minutes

Ingredients

- 2 salmon fillets
- 1 tbsp duck fat
- Salt and black pepper to taste
- 2 tbsp butter
- ½ tsp tarragon
- ¼ cup heavy cream

Directions:

1. Season the salmon with salt and pepper.
2. Melt the duck fat in a pan. Set it over medium heat. Add salmon and cook for 4 minutes on both sides; set aside. Into that, melt the butter and add the tarragon.
3. Cook for 30 seconds to infuse the flavors.
4. Whisk in heavy cream and cook for a minute.
5. Serve salmon topped with the sauce.

Nutritional Value (Per Serving): Cal 468; Net Carbs 1.5g; Fat 40g; Protein 22g

Crab Cakes

Servings: 8

Cooking Time: 15 minutes

Ingredients

- 2 tbsp coconut oil
- 1 tbsp lemon juice
- 1 cup lump crab meat
- 2 tbsp parsley
- 2 tsp Dijon mustard
- 1 egg, beaten
- 1 ½ tbsp coconut flour
- Salt and black pepper to taste

Directions:

1. Place crab meat in a bowl. Add the remaining ingredients, except for coconut oil.

2. Mix well to combine. Make 8 crab cakes out of the mixture.

3. Melt the oil in a skillet.

4. Add the crab cakes and cook for 2-3 minutes per side.

Nutritional Value (Per Serving): Cal 65; Net Carbs 3.6g; Fat 5g; Protein 5.3g

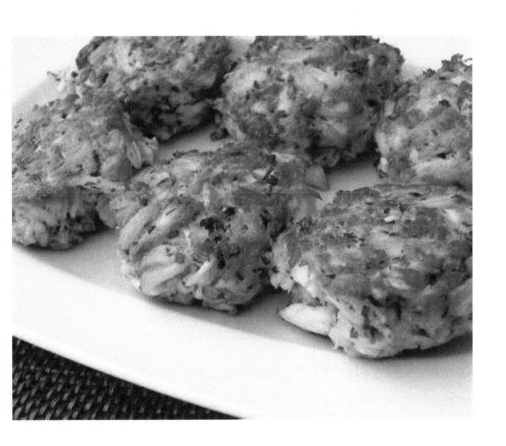

Spicy Sea Bass with Hazelnuts

Servings: 2

Cooking Time: 20 minutes

Ingredients

- 2 sea bass fillets
- 2 tbsp butter
- ⅓ cup roasted hazelnuts
- A pinch of cayenne pepper

Directions:

1. Preheat your oven to 425° F. Line a baking dish with waxed paper.

2. Melt the butter and brush it over the fish. Process the cayenne pepper and hazelnuts in a food processor to achieve a smooth consistency.

3. Coat the sea bass with the hazelnut mixture.

4. Place in the oven and bake for about minutes.

Nutritional Value (Per Serving): Kcal 467, Fat: 31g, Net Carbs: 2.8g, Protein: 40g

VEGETABLES

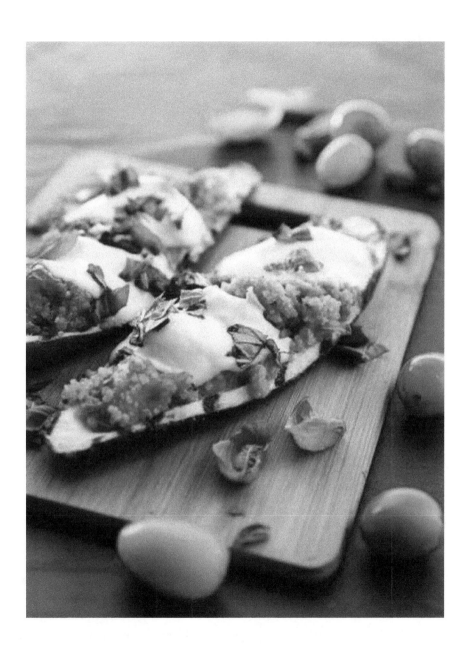

Vegetarian Chili with Avocado Cream

Preparation Time: 15 minutes

Cooking Time: 25 minutes

Servings: 8

Ingredients:

- tablespoons olive oil
- 1/2 onion, finely chopped
- 1 tablespoon minced garlic
- 2 jalapeño peppers, chopped
- 1 red bell pepper, diced
- 1 teaspoon ground cumin
- 2 tablespoons chili powder
- 2 cups pecans, chopped
- 4 cups canned diced tomatoes and their juice

Topping:

- cup sour cream
- 1 avocado, diced
- tablespoons fresh cilantro, chopped

Directions:

1. Heat olive oil.

2. Toss in the onion, garlic, jalapeño peppers, and red bell pepper, then sauté for about 4 minutes until tender.

3. Put in the chili powder and cumin and stir for 30 seconds.

4. Fold in the pecans, tomatoes, and their juice, then bring to a boil.

5. Simmer uncovered for about 20 minutes to infuse the flavors, stirring occasionally.

6. Remove from the heat to eight bowls.

7. Evenly top each bowl of chili with sour cream, diced avocado, and fresh cilantro.

Nutritional Value:

Calories: 318 Fat: 14.4g Fiber: 17.5g Carbohydrates: 9.5 g Protein: 14g

Cherry Tomato Gratin

Preparation Time: 15 minutes

Cooking Time: 20 minutes

Servings: 4

Ingredients:

- 2 tablespoons olive oil,
- 1/2 cup cherry tomatoes halved
- 1/2 cup mayonnaise, Keto-friendly
- 1/2 cup vegan Mozzarella cheese, cut into pieces
- 1 ounce (28 g) vegan Parmesan cheese, shredded
- 1 tablespoon basil pesto
- Pepper and salt
- 1 cup watercress

Directions:

1. Let the oven heat up to 400F. Grease a baking pan with olive oil.

2. Combine the cherry tomatoes, mayo, vegan Mozzarella cheese, 1/2 ounce (14 g) of Parmesan cheese, basil pesto, salt, and black pepper baking pan. Scatter with the remaining Parmesan.

3. Baking time: 20 minutes.

4. Remove them from the oven and divide them among four plates. Top with watercress and olive oil, and slice to serve.

Nutritional Value:

Calories: 254 Fat: 12.1g Fiber: 9.3g Carbohydrates: 11.1g Protein: 9.5g

Stuffed Zucchini

Preparation Time: 20 minutes

Cooking Time: 20 minutes

Servings: 4

Ingredients:

- 4 medium zucchinis, halved lengthwise
- 1 cup red bell pepper, seeded and minced
- 1/2 cup Kalamata olives, pitted and minced
- 1/2 cup fresh tomatoes, minced
- 1 teaspoon garlic, minced
- tablespoon dried oregano, crushed
- Salt and ground black pepper, as required
- 1/2 cup feta cheese, crumbled

Directions:

1. Grease a large baking sheet.
2. With a melon baller, scoop out the flesh of each zucchini half. Discard the flesh.
3. In a bowl, mix the bell pepper, olives, tomatoes, garlic, oregano, salt, and black pepper.
4. Stuff each zucchini half with the veggie mixture evenly.
5. Arrange zucchini halves onto the prepared baking sheet and bake for about 15 minutes.
6. Now, set the oven to broiler on high.

7. Top each zucchini half with feta cheese and broil for about 3 minutes. Serve hot.

Nutritional Value:

Calories: 314 Fat: 12.4g Fiber: 9.4g Carbohydrates: 4.1 g Protein: 7.4g

Sweet & Spicy Carrots

Preparation Time: 18 minutes

Servings: 4

Ingredients:

- 1 pound quartered lengthwise and halved carrots
- 1 tbsp. Erythritol
- 2 tbsp. butter
- 3 tsp ground mustard
- 1 tsp ground cumin
- ½ tsp cayenne pepper
- ¼ tsp red pepper flakes
- Salt and freshly ground black pepper, to taste
- 1/8 tsp ground cinnamon

Directions:

1. In the bottom of the Instant Pot, arrange a steamer basket and pour 1 cup of water.
2. Place the carrots into the steamer basket.
3. Secure the lid and place the pressure valve in the "Seal" position.
4. Select "Manual" and cook under "High Pressure" for about 1 minute.
5. Select the "Cancel" and carefully do a "Quick" release.
6. Remove the lid and transfer the carrots to a bowl.
7. Remove water from the pot and with paper towels, pat dry.

8. Select the "Sauté" mode for Power Pressure Cooker. In the pot of the Pressure Cooker, melt butter and stir in the remaining ingredients.

9. Stir in the carrots and cook for about 1 minute.

10. Select the "Cancel" and serve warm with the sprinkling of cinnamon.

Nutritional Value:

Calories 112, Total Fat 6.6g, Net Carbs 3.50g, Protein 1.7g, Fiber 3.3g

Bell Pepper Gumbo

Preparation Time: 20 minutes

Servings: 3

Ingredients:

- tbsp. olive oil
- 4 minced garlic cloves
- ½ tsp cumin seeds
- 1 seeded and cut into long strips green bell pepper
- 1 seeded and cut into long strips red bell pepper
- 1 seeded and cut into long strips yellow bell pepper
- 1 seeded and cut into long strips bell pepper
- ½ tsp red chili powder
- ¼ tsp ground turmeric
- Salt and freshly ground black pepper, to taste ¼ cup water
- ½ tbsp. fresh lemon juice

Directions:

1. Place the oil in the Instant Pot and select "Sauté." Then add the garlic and cumin and cook for about 1 minute.

2. Select the "Cancel" and stir in the remaining ingredients except for lemon juice.

3. Secure the lid and place the pressure valve in the "Seal" position.

4. Select "Manual" and cook under "High Pressure" for about 2 minutes.

5. Select the "Cancel" and carefully do a "Quick" release.

6. Remove the lid and select "Sauté."

7. Stir in lemon juice and cook for about 1-2 minutes.

8. Select the "Cancel" and serve.

Nutritional Value:

Calories 101, Total Fat 5.3g, Net Carbs 4.6g, Protein 2g, Fiber 2.5g

Provincial Ratatouille

Preparation Time: 26 minutes

Servings: 6

Ingredients:

- 1 sliced into thin circles large zucchini
- 1 sliced into thin circles medium eggplant
- 2 sliced into thin disks medium tomatoes
- 1 sliced into thin circles small yellow onion
- 1 tbsp. dried thyme -divided
- Salt and freshly ground black pepper, to taste
- 2 finely chopped large garlic cloves
- 2 tbsp. olive oil
- 1 tbsp. apple cider vinegar
- 1 cup of water

Directions:

1. In a bowl, add all vegetables and sprinkle with half of the thyme, salt, and black pepper.
2. In the bottom of a foil-lined round springform pan, spread some garlic.
3. Layer the vegetables into a tight snail-like circle over the garlic, alternating between eggplant, zucchini, onion, and tomato slices. -Keep the slices close together, overlapping slightly.

4. Sprinkle with the remaining garlic, thyme, salt, and black pepper, and drizzle with oil and vinegar.

5. In the bottom of the Instant Pot, arrange a steamer trivet and pour 1 cup of water.

6. Place the pan on top of the trivet.

7. Secure the lid and place the pressure valve in the "Seal" position.

8. Select "Manual" and cook under "Low Pressure" for about 6 minutes.

9. Select the "Cancel" and carefully do a "Natural" release for about 6 minutes and then do a "Quick" release.

10. Remove the lid and transfer the pan to a counter.

11. Carefully, transfer the veggie mixture onto serving plates and serve.

Nutrition Values:

Calories 86, Total Fat 5.1g, Net Carbs 1.7g, Protein 2.1g, Fiber 4.4g

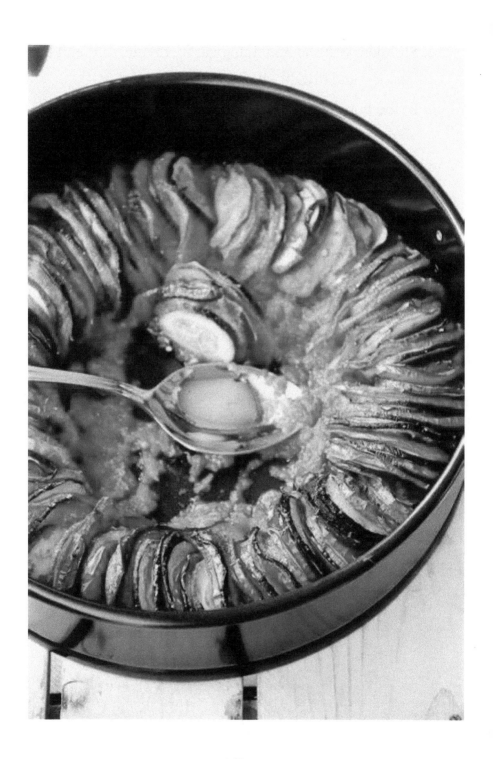

DESSERT

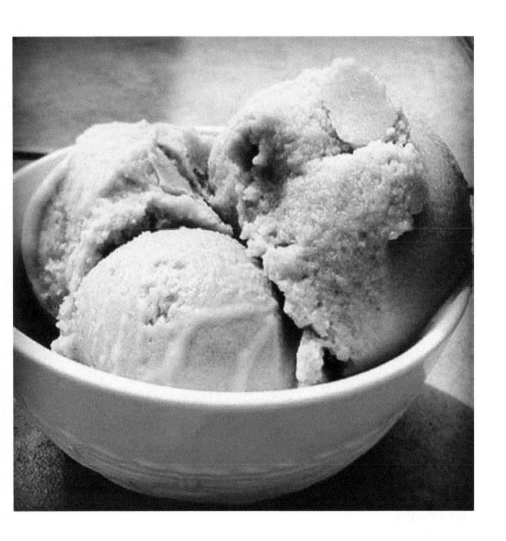

Coconut Cheesecake

Preparation Time: 15 minutes

Cooking Time: 25 minutes

Servings: 12

Ingredients:

Crust:

- egg whites
- 1/4 cup erythritol
- cups desiccated coconut
- 1 tsp. coconut oil
- 1/4 cup melted butter

Filling:

- 3 tbsp. lemon juice
- 6 ounces raspberries
- 2 cups erythritol
- 1 cup whipped cream
- Zest of 1 lemon
- 24 ounces cream cheese

Directions:

1. Line the pan with parchment paper. Preheat oven to 350°F and mix all crust ingredients.

2. Pour the crust into the pan. Bake for about 25 minutes; let cool. Whisk the cream cheese in a container.

3. Add the lemon juice, zest, and erythritol. Fold in whipped cream mixture.

4. Fold in the raspberries gently. Spoon the filling into the crust. Place in the fridge for 4 hours.

Nutritional Value:

Calories: 214 Fat: 11.4g Fiber: 8.4g Carbohydrates: 5.4g Protein: 9.1g

Cashew and Raspberry Truffles

Preparation Time: 10 minutes

Cooking Time: 0 minutes

Servings: 4

Ingredients:

- 2 cups raw cashews
- 2 tbsp. flax seed
- 1 1/2 cups sugar-free raspberry preserves
- 3 tbsp. swerve
- 10 oz unsweetened chocolate chips
- 3 tbsp. olive oil

Directions:

1. Grind the cashews and flax seeds in a blender for 45 seconds until smoothly crushed; add the raspberry and 2 tbsp. of swerve.

2. Process further for 1 minute until well combined. Form 1-inch balls of the mixture, place on the baking sheet, and freeze for 1 hour or until firmed up.

3. Melt the chocolate chips, oil, and 1tbsp. of swerve in a microwave for 1 1/2 minute.

4. Toss the truffles to coat in the chocolate mixture, put on the baking sheet, and freeze further for at least 2 hours

Nutritional Value:

Calories: 199 Fat: 4.1g Fiber: 3.1g Carbohydrates: 1 g Protein: 3.2g

Black Bean Brownies

Preparation Time: 15 minutes

Cooking Time: 25 minutes

Servings: 12

Ingredients:

- 1 15-oz can of black beans
- 2 large flax eggs
- 3 tablespoon of coconut oil
- 3/4 cup cocoa powder
- 1/4 tablespoon of salt
- 1 tablespoon pure vanilla extract
- 1/2 cup of organic cane sugar
- 1 1/2 tablespoon of baking powder

Toppings:

- Crushed walnuts
- Pecans
- Daily-free semisweet chocolate chips

Directions:

1. Let the oven heat to 350F.prepare a baking dish lined with parchment paper.
2. Get a 12-slot standard size muffin pot and grease. Rinse your black beans well and drain.
3. Get the bowl of a food processor and prepare flax egg

4. Leave out walnuts and other toppings and add the remaining ingredients and puree

5. Get the muffin tin and pour the batter into it. Ensure that the top is smooth

6. Bake the batter until the tops are dry and the edges start to pull away from the sides. This lasts 25 minutes.

7. Remove the pan and let it cool. Serve and enjoy!

Nutritional Value:

Calories: 259 Fat: 12.1g Fiber: 10.9g Carbohydrates: 3.8 g Protein: 5.1g

Vanilla Flan

Preparation Time: 15 minutes

Cooking Time: 60 minutes

Servings: 4

Ingredients:

- 1/3 cup erythritol, for caramel
- 2 cups almond milk
- 4 eggs
- 1 tbsp. vanilla extract
- 1 tbsp. lemon zest
- 1/2 cup erythritol, for custard
- 2 cup heavy whipping cream
- Mint leaves, to serve

Directions:

1. Heat erythritol for the caramel in a deep pan. Add 2-3 tablespoons of water, and bring to a boil. Reduce the heat and cook until the caramel turns golden brown.

2. Divide between 4-6 metal tins. Set aside to cool.

3. In a bowl, mix eggs, remaining erythritol, lemon zest, and vanilla. Add almond milk and beat until well combined.

4. Pour the custard into each caramel-lined ramekin and place it in a deep baking tin.

5. Fill over the way with the remaining hot water. Bake at 345°F for 45-50 minutes.

6. Take out the ramekins and let cool for at least 4 hours in the fridge.

7. Run a knife slowly around the edges to invert onto a dish. Serve with dollops of whipped cream, scattered with mint leaves.

Nutritional Value:

Calories: 231 Fat: 10.3g Fiber: 4.1g Carbohydrates: 1.2 g Protein: 3.7g

Key Lime Truffles

Servings: 6

Cooking Time: 5 minutes

Ingredients

- ¼ cup cocoa powder mixed with 2 tbsp swerve sugar
- 1 cup dark chocolate, chopped
- 2/3 cup heavy cream
- 2 tsp lime extract

Directions:

1. Heat heavy cream in a pan over low heat until tiny bubbles form around the pan's edges. Turn the heat off. Pour dark chocolate into the pan, swirl the pan to allow the hot cream to spread over the chocolate, and then gently stir the mixture until smooth. Mix in lime extract and transfer to a bowl.

2. Refrigerate for 4 hours. Line 2 baking trays with parchment papers; set one aside and pour cocoa powder mixture onto the other. Take out the chocolate mixture; form bite-size balls out of the mix and roll all round in the cocoa powder to completely coat. Place the truffles on the baking tray and refrigerate for 30 minutes before Serves.

Nutritional Value (Per Serving):

Cal 143; Net Carbs 0.6g, Fat 12g, Protein 2.4g

Lime Avocado Ice Cream

Servings: 4

Cooking Time: 10 minutes

Ingredients

- 2 large avocados, pitted
- Juice and zest of 3 limes
- 1/3 cup erythritol
- 1¾ cups coconut cream
- ¼ tsp vanilla extract

Directions:

1. In a blender, combine avocado pulp, lime juice and zest, erythritol, coconut cream, and vanilla extract. Process until smooth.

2. Pour the mixture into an ice cream maker and freeze.

3. When ready, remove and scoop the ice cream into bowls. Serve immediately.

Nutritional Value (Per Serving): Cal 260; Net Carbs 4g; Fat 25g; Protein 4g

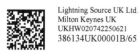

Lightning Source UK Ltd.
Milton Keynes UK
UKHW020742250621
386134UK00001B/65

9 781803 176765